I0106333

This publication is intended to provide educational information for the reader on the covered subjects. It is not intended to take the place of personalized medical counseling, diagnosis, and treatment from a trained healthcare professional.

ISBN 978-1-998740-05-5 (Paperback)
ISBN 978-1-998740-06-2 (eBook)

Printed and bound in USA
Published by Loons Press

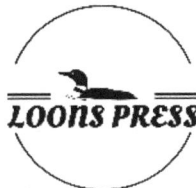

LOONS PRESS

Table Of Contents

Chapter 1   **7**

Understanding Frailty   **7**

   The Definition of Frailty   7

   The Causes of Frailty   10

   The Impact of Frailty on Health and
Quality of Life   13

Chapter 2   **18**

The Importance of Strength Training   **18**

   What is Strength Training?   18

   Benefits of Strength Training for Older
Adults   21

   Overcoming Barriers to Starting
Strength Training   24

Chapter 3   **29**

Nutrition for Strength and Vitality   **29**

   Essential Nutrients for Muscle Health   29

   Meal Planning Tips for Older Adults   32

   Supplements: Do You Need Them?   34

Chapter 4   **39**

Creating a Safe Exercise Environment   **39**

Assessing Your Home for Safety   39

Choosing the Right Equipment   42

Finding the Right Space for Exercise   44

Chapter 5   **48**

Developing a Personalized Strength Training Program   **48**

Assessing Your Current Fitness Level   48

Setting Realistic Goals   51

Types of Strength Training Exercises   54

Chapter 6   **58**

Incorporating Flexibility and Balance Training   **58**

The Role of Flexibility in Preventing Frailty   58

Balance Exercises to Reduce Fall Risk   61

Combining Flexibility and Strength Training   64

Chapter 7   **68**

The Role of Social Connections   **68**

     Building a Support Network   68

     Group Activities and Classes   71

     The Psychological Benefits of Social Interaction   73

Chapter 8   **78**

Monitoring Progress and Staying Motivated   **78**

     Tracking Your Strength Gains   78

     Adjusting Your Program as You Progress   81

     Celebrating Milestones   83

Chapter 9   **88**

Overcoming Challenges and Setbacks   **88**

     Common Obstacles to Strength Training   88

     Strategies for Staying on Track   91

     Dealing with Injuries and Recovery   94

Chapter 10   **98**

Maintaining Long-Term Strength and Health   **98**

Making Strength Training a Lifelong Habit   98

Adapting Your Routine as You Age   101

The Future of Aging: Trends in Strength and Health   103

Chapter 11   **108**

Resources for Further Learning   **108**

Recommended Books and Articles   108

Online Courses and Videos   111

Local Community Resources and Programs   114

Author Notes & Acknowledgments   **118**

Author Bio   **120**

How To Prevent Frailty

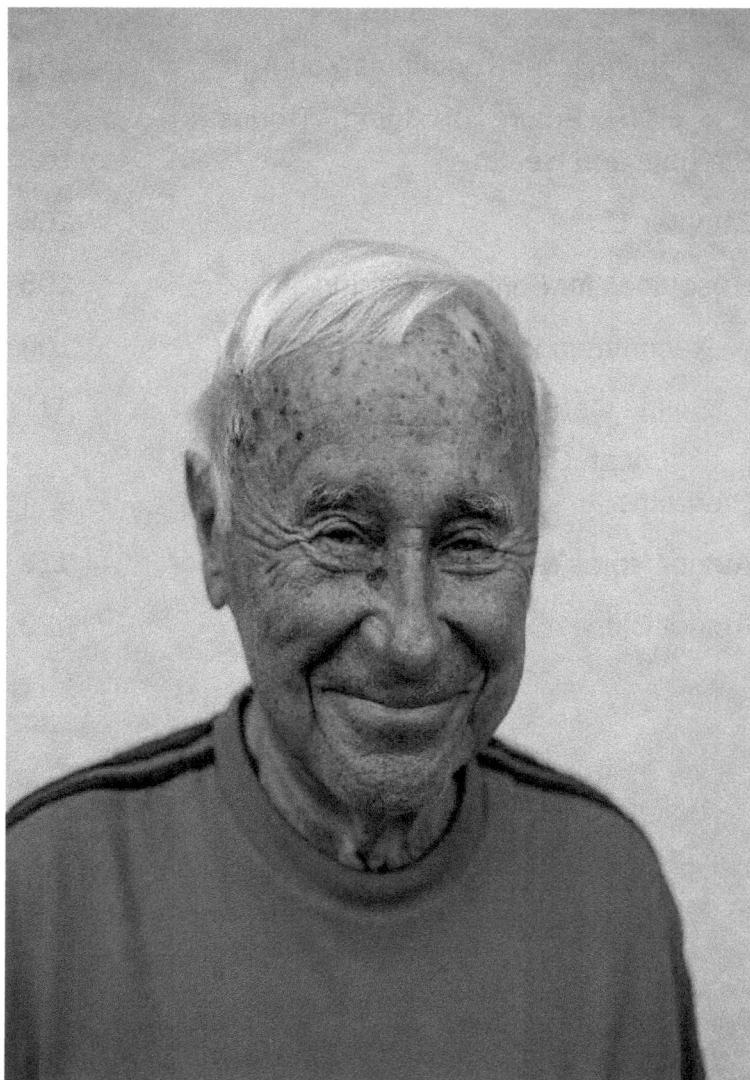

Chapter 1

Understanding Frailty

The Definition of Frailty

Frailty is a complex and multifaceted condition that primarily affects older adults, characterized by a decrease in physiological reserve and increased vulnerability to stressors.

It is often described as a clinical syndrome that encompasses a range of physical, emotional, and social factors.

The most common definition of frailty includes a combination of weakness, weight loss, exhaustion, low physical activity, and slow walking speed. Understanding this definition is crucial for individuals who wish to prevent frailty, as it highlights the key areas that can be targeted for improvement.

The physical dimension of frailty is particularly significant. As individuals age, muscle mass and strength tend to decline, which can lead to difficulties in performing daily activities. This loss of strength and mobility can create a cycle where decreased activity leads to further deterioration.

Recognizing the signs of physical frailty, such as difficulty standing up from a seated position or climbing stairs, is essential for early intervention. Engaging in regular strength training and physical activity can help mitigate these effects, ultimately enhancing overall resilience.

Emotional and psychological factors also play a critical role in defining frailty. Depression, anxiety, and social isolation can exacerbate physical decline and increase the risk of frailty.

The interplay between mental health and physical capabilities means that addressing psychological well-being is as important as promoting physical fitness.

Activities that foster social engagement and mental stimulation can contribute to a holistic approach to preventing frailty, emphasizing the importance of nurturing both body and mind.

Another key element in the definition of frailty is the impact of chronic diseases. Conditions such as diabetes, heart disease, and arthritis can significantly affect an individual's overall health and contribute to frailty.

Managing these diseases effectively through regular medical check-ups, medication adherence, and lifestyle modifications is crucial for reducing the risk of frailty. Individuals should be proactive in their healthcare, seeking guidance from medical professionals to tailor strategies that address their specific health needs.

In summary, frailty is a multifaceted condition that encompasses physical, emotional, and chronic health factors. By understanding its definition, individuals can identify the signs and take actionable steps to prevent frailty.

Prioritizing physical activity, addressing mental health, and managing chronic conditions are all integral parts of a comprehensive approach. This understanding lays the foundation for a proactive lifestyle that not only aims to prevent frailty but also promotes overall well-being as one ages.

The Causes of Frailty

Frailty is a complex syndrome characterized by a decline in physiological reserve and increased vulnerability to stressors. Understanding the causes of frailty is essential for prevention and management. One of the primary contributors to frailty is the natural aging process.

As individuals age, biological changes occur, including a decrease in muscle mass, strength, and endurance. This process, known as sarcopenia, significantly impacts mobility and functionality, making older adults more susceptible to falls, injuries, and overall decline in health.

Chronic diseases are another significant factor leading to frailty. Conditions such as diabetes, heart disease, and chronic obstructive pulmonary disease (COPD) can contribute to a downward spiral of health. These illnesses can result in decreased physical activity and energy levels, exacerbating muscle loss and functional decline.

The interplay between chronic disease and frailty creates a cycle that can be difficult to break, making it imperative for individuals to manage their health proactively through regular medical check-ups and lifestyle modifications.

Nutritional deficiencies also play a critical role in the development of frailty. As people age, their dietary needs change, and many may not consume enough essential nutrients, such as protein, vitamins, and minerals. Inadequate nutrition can lead to muscle weakness and a compromised immune system, further increasing vulnerability to health issues.

Addressing these deficiencies through a balanced diet rich in whole foods can help mitigate the risk of frailty and promote overall well-being.

Psychosocial factors, including social isolation and depression, can contribute significantly to frailty. Older adults who experience loneliness or lack social support may engage in less physical activity, leading to a decline in physical health.

Mental health issues can also reduce motivation and energy levels, making it challenging to maintain an active lifestyle. Encouraging social engagement and mental health support can be vital in preventing the onset of frailty among older adults.

Lastly, environmental factors, such as living conditions and access to healthcare, can influence the risk of frailty. Poor housing, limited access to nutritious food, and inadequate healthcare services can all contribute to a decline in physical and mental health. Creating supportive environments that promote active living, social connections, and access to healthcare resources is essential in combating frailty.

By addressing these multifaceted causes, individuals can take proactive steps toward maintaining strength and vitality as they age.

The Impact of Frailty on Health and Quality of Life

Frailty is a syndrome characterized by a decline in physiological reserve and increased vulnerability to stressors. Its impact on health is profound, as frail individuals often experience multiple comorbidities that can complicate treatment and significantly impair their ability to function.

This decline is not merely a consequence of aging but a multifaceted issue that can stem from factors such as malnutrition, sedentary lifestyle, and chronic diseases. Understanding how frailty affects health is crucial for individuals seeking to prevent this condition, as it highlights the importance of proactive measures in maintaining physical and mental well-being.

The physical deterioration commonly associated with frailty can lead to a cascade of health problems. Weakness, weight loss, exhaustion, and reduced physical activity are hallmark signs that can hinder mobility and increase the risk of falls and injuries.

Moreover, frail individuals often find it challenging to recover from illnesses or surgeries, resulting in longer hospital stays and a heightened risk of complications. This interconnectedness of health issues emphasizes the need for regular health assessments and interventions that focus on strength training and nutritional support to mitigate these risks.

Frailty also has a significant impact on mental health and quality of life. Individuals grappling with frailty may experience feelings of helplessness, anxiety, and depression due to their declining physical capabilities and the loss of independence.

Social isolation is another common consequence, as frail individuals may withdraw from activities and relationships that once brought them joy. This decline in mental health can create a vicious cycle, further exacerbating physical frailty and leading to a decrease in overall life satisfaction. Addressing these psychological aspects is essential when developing strategies to prevent frailty.

The quality of life for frail individuals often diminishes as they face limitations in daily activities and social participation. Simple tasks, such as grocery shopping or attending social events, can become daunting challenges, leading to a sedentary lifestyle that perpetuates frailty.

Furthermore, the inability to engage in meaningful activities can result in a diminished sense of purpose, which is crucial for emotional well-being. By promoting physical activity, social engagement, and mental stimulation, individuals can significantly enhance their quality of life and reduce the impact of frailty.

Preventing frailty requires a comprehensive approach that considers both physical and mental health. Engaging in regular exercise, particularly strength training, can counteract muscle weakness and improve balance, thus reducing the risk of falls.

Adequate nutrition, focusing on a balanced diet rich in protein and essential nutrients, is equally important in maintaining health and vitality.

Additionally, fostering social connections and engaging in community activities can enhance emotional well-being and combat feelings of isolation. By addressing these various aspects of health and quality of life, individuals can take proactive steps toward preventing frailty and ensuring a healthier, more fulfilling aging process.

How To Prevent Frailty

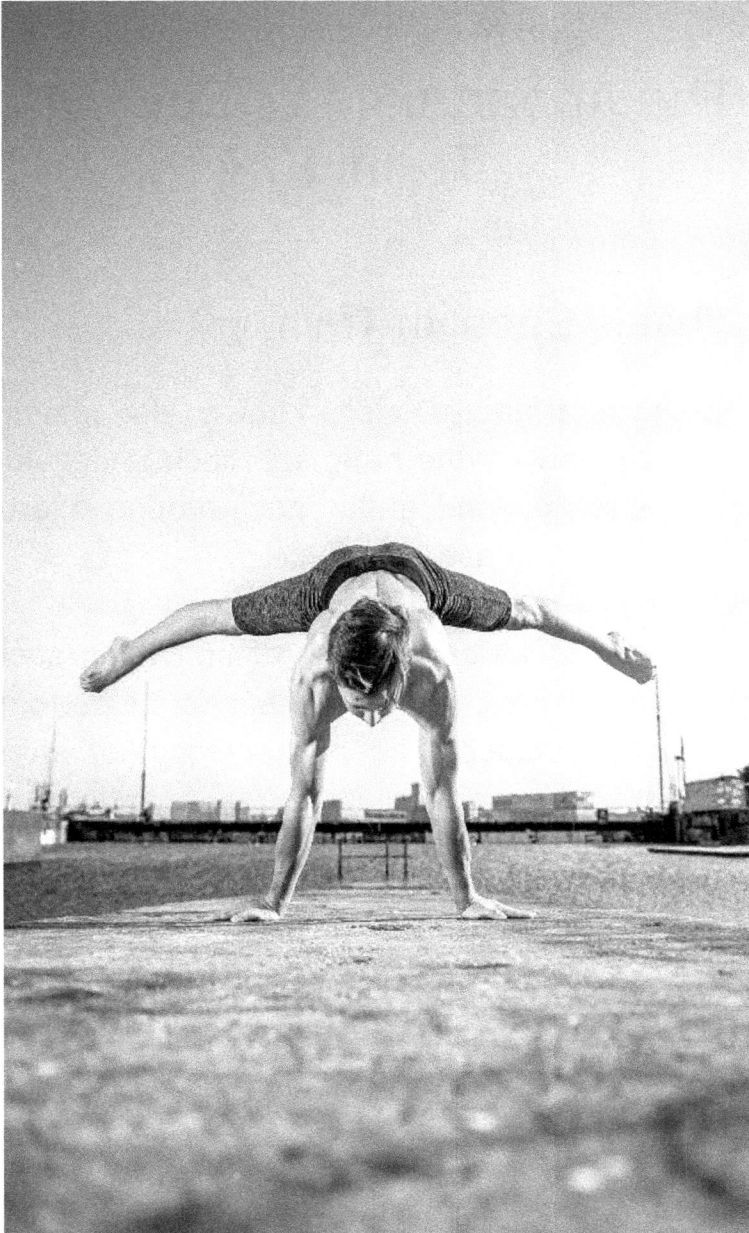

Building Strength as You Age

Chapter 2

The Importance of Strength Training

What is Strength Training?

Strength training, also known as resistance training, involves a systematic approach to developing muscular strength and endurance through exercises that exert force against resistance.

This can include a variety of activities, such as lifting weights, using resistance bands, or performing bodyweight exercises. The primary goal of strength training is to increase muscle mass and strength, which can significantly benefit individuals as they age.

By engaging in regular strength training, older adults can counteract the natural loss of muscle mass and strength that occurs due to aging, a condition known as sarcopenia.

One of the most critical aspects of strength training is its impact on overall health. Engaging in resistance exercises not only builds muscle but also enhances bone density, improves joint function, and increases metabolism.

These benefits are particularly important for older adults, as maintaining bone density helps reduce the risk of fractures and osteoporosis, while improved joint function can lead to better mobility and reduced risk of falls. Furthermore, a higher metabolic rate contributes to weight management, which is crucial for overall health and well-being.

Strength training also plays a vital role in enhancing functional fitness, which is the ability to perform everyday activities with ease. As individuals age, they may find routine tasks such as climbing stairs, lifting groceries, or standing up from a seated position more challenging.

By incorporating strength training into their routine, older adults can improve their functional strength, making these activities more manageable. This increased ability to perform daily tasks not only boosts confidence but also promotes independence, reducing the likelihood of frailty and its associated risks.

In addition to the physical benefits, strength training can have significant psychological advantages. Engaging in regular exercise, including resistance training, has been shown to reduce symptoms of anxiety and depression, improve mood, and enhance overall mental well-being.

For older adults, maintaining a positive mental state is essential for quality of life. The sense of accomplishment that comes from achieving strength training goals can also foster a sense of empowerment, motivating individuals to stay active and engaged in their health journey.

To get started with strength training, individuals do not need to invest in expensive gym memberships or equipment. Many effective exercises can be performed at home using body weight or minimal equipment, such as resistance bands or dumbbells. It is crucial, however, to approach strength training with proper guidance to ensure safety and effectiveness.

Consulting with a healthcare professional or a certified trainer can help create a tailored program that considers individual health conditions and fitness levels, paving the way for a successful journey toward preventing frailty through strength training.

Benefits of Strength Training for Older Adults

Strength training offers numerous benefits for older adults, particularly in the context of preventing frailty. As individuals age, they often experience a natural decline in muscle mass and strength, known as sarcopenia. Engaging in regular strength training can counteract this decline, helping older adults maintain and even increase their muscle mass.

This is crucial not only for physical appearance but also for functional independence. By building and preserving muscle, older adults can perform daily activities with greater ease, enhancing their overall quality of life.

In addition to preserving muscle mass, strength training plays a significant role in improving bone density. Osteoporosis, a condition characterized by weak and brittle bones, is a common concern among older adults. Resistance exercises stimulate bone growth and can help prevent or slow the progression of bone density loss.

This is particularly important for older women, who are at a higher risk of developing osteoporosis after menopause. By incorporating strength training into their routines, older adults can promote stronger bones and reduce their risk of fractures.

Strength training also contributes to enhanced balance and coordination, which are critical factors in fall prevention. Falls are a leading cause of injury among older adults, often resulting in severe consequences such as broken bones or loss of independence.

Through strength training, older adults can improve their core strength and stability, which are essential for maintaining balance. Exercises that focus on the lower body, such as squats and lunges, can significantly reduce the risk of falls, allowing older adults to navigate their environment more safely.

Moreover, the psychological benefits of strength training should not be overlooked. Regular physical activity, including strength training, has been shown to reduce symptoms of anxiety and depression, which can be prevalent among older adults.

The sense of accomplishment that comes from setting and achieving fitness goals can boost self-esteem and promote a positive outlook on life. Additionally, participating in group strength training classes fosters social connections, further enhancing mental well-being.

Finally, strength training can lead to improved metabolic health. As individuals age, their metabolism tends to slow down, increasing the risk of weight gain and associated health issues such as diabetes and cardiovascular diseases.

Strength training helps to increase muscle mass, which in turn elevates resting metabolic rate. This means that even at rest, individuals who engage in strength training burn more calories. By incorporating strength training into their routines, older adults can better manage their weight and reduce the risk of chronic diseases, contributing to their overall health and longevity.

Overcoming Barriers to Starting Strength Training

Overcoming barriers to starting strength training is essential for individuals seeking to prevent frailty as they age. Many people face a variety of obstacles that can deter them from engaging in regular strength training, including physical limitations, lack of knowledge, and psychological factors.

Identifying these barriers is the first step in creating a tailored approach that promotes a sustainable and effective strength training routine.

By acknowledging these challenges, individuals can better equip themselves to take actionable steps toward improving their physical health.

One common barrier is the fear of injury, particularly among older adults. Many individuals may have experienced past injuries or have chronic conditions that make them wary of engaging in physical activity. It is crucial to address these concerns by emphasizing the importance of starting with low-impact exercises and gradually increasing intensity.

Consulting with healthcare professionals or certified trainers can also provide individuals with personalized guidance and reassurance. Education on proper form and techniques can significantly reduce the risk of injury, allowing individuals to build confidence in their abilities and engage more fully in strength training.

Another barrier is the misconception that strength training is only for young or athletic individuals. This stereotype can discourage older adults from participating in these beneficial exercises. It is important to highlight that strength training is not only accessible but also highly beneficial for individuals of all ages.

Research has shown that even light resistance training can lead to significant improvements in muscle strength, balance, and overall well-being for older adults. By showcasing success stories and providing relatable examples, individuals can be motivated to see strength training as a vital component of their health and fitness journey.

Time constraints often serve as a significant barrier for many people. Busy lifestyles can make it challenging to fit in regular workouts. However, strength training does not have to require extensive time commitments. Short, efficient workouts can be designed to fit even the most hectic schedules.

Emphasizing the flexibility of strength training, such as performing exercises at home or incorporating them into daily routines, can help individuals find opportunities for physical activity. Simple strategies, like setting aside just 20-30 minutes a few times a week, can lead to meaningful gains in strength and health.

Finally, psychological barriers, such as lack of motivation or feelings of inadequacy, can hinder the initiation of strength training. Individuals may doubt their ability to perform exercises correctly or fear judgment in a gym setting. Building a supportive community can play a crucial role in overcoming these barriers. Engaging in group classes or finding a workout buddy can provide encouragement and accountability.

Additionally, setting realistic goals and celebrating small achievements can foster a sense of accomplishment and motivation. By addressing psychological factors and creating an environment conducive to growth, individuals can cultivate a more positive relationship with strength training and its role in preventing frailty.

How To Prevent Frailty

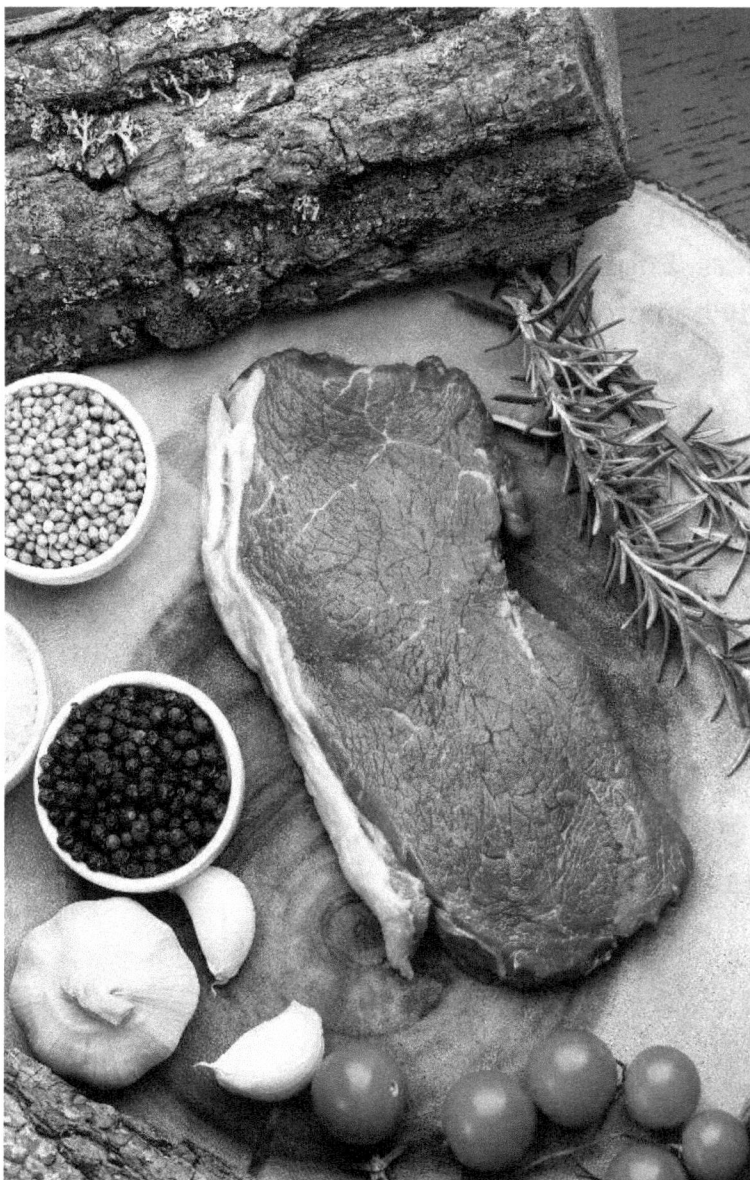

Chapter 3

Nutrition for Strength and Vitality

Essential Nutrients for Muscle Health

Essential nutrients play a crucial role in maintaining muscle health, especially as we age. As individuals seek to prevent frailty, understanding these nutrients becomes vital. Protein is the cornerstone of muscle maintenance and growth.

It provides the building blocks, known as amino acids, necessary for muscle repair and regeneration. Older adults often require higher protein intake to counteract the natural decline in muscle mass that occurs with aging.

Sources of high-quality protein include lean meats, fish, dairy products, legumes, and nuts, which can all help promote muscle health and overall strength.

In addition to protein, essential fatty acids are significant for muscle health. Omega-3 fatty acids, in particular, have been shown to help reduce muscle inflammation, enhance muscle protein synthesis, and improve overall muscle function. These fatty acids can be found in fatty fish such as salmon and mackerel, as well as in flaxseeds and walnuts. Including these sources in one's diet can contribute to better muscle maintenance and recovery, helping to mitigate the effects of aging on muscle tissue.

Vitamins and minerals also play a pivotal role in supporting muscle health. Vitamin D, for instance, is essential for calcium absorption and muscle function. Deficiency in vitamin D can lead to muscle weakness and increased risk of falls, which are particularly concerning for older adults.

Furthermore, minerals such as calcium and magnesium are critical for muscle contractions and overall muscle performance. Ensuring an adequate intake of these vitamins and minerals through a balanced diet or supplements can significantly enhance muscle strength and reduce the risk of frailty.

Hydration is another essential factor that often gets overlooked in discussions about muscle health. Proper hydration is necessary for maintaining optimal muscle function, as even mild dehydration can impair performance and increase the risk of cramps and fatigue.

Older adults may be more susceptible to dehydration due to changes in thirst perception and kidney function, making it crucial to prioritize fluid intake. Water, herbal teas, and hydrating fruits and vegetables can help maintain hydration levels and support muscle health.

Lastly, it is important to recognize that the synergistic effect of these essential nutrients contributes to overall muscle health. A well-rounded diet that incorporates adequate protein, healthy fats, vitamins, minerals, and hydration will create a solid foundation for muscle maintenance and strength. As individuals strive to prevent frailty, focusing on these nutrients and making conscious dietary choices can lead to improved muscle function, enhanced mobility, and a better quality of life as they age.

Meal Planning Tips for Older Adults

Meal planning is a crucial aspect for older adults aiming to maintain their health and prevent frailty. A well-structured meal plan not only ensures that nutritional needs are met but also helps in managing weight, boosting energy levels, and enhancing overall well-being. When creating a meal plan, it is essential to consider the unique dietary requirements that come with aging, such as increased need for protein, fiber, vitamins, and minerals, while also being mindful of any food restrictions due to health conditions.

Incorporating a variety of foods into the weekly meal plan can help prevent nutritional deficiencies and keep meals interesting. Older adults should focus on whole foods, including fruits, vegetables, whole grains, lean proteins, and healthy fats.

Aim for a colorful plate, as different colors often represent different nutrients. For instance, dark leafy greens provide iron and calcium, while orange vegetables are rich in beta-carotene. Planning meals that include diverse food groups can enhance nutrient intake and improve dietary satisfaction.

Portion control is another essential element in meal planning for older adults. As metabolism slows with age, it is vital to be aware of portion sizes to avoid unnecessary weight gain. Using smaller plates can help control portions while still allowing for a visually satisfying meal. Additionally, older adults may benefit from eating smaller, more frequent meals throughout the day rather than a few large ones. This approach can aid digestion, maintain stable energy levels, and prevent feelings of hunger, which can lead to poor food choices.

Preparation methods also play a significant role in meal planning. Opting for cooking methods that preserve nutrients, such as steaming, baking, or grilling, can enhance the health benefits of meals. It is advisable to limit frying and heavy sauces that can add unnecessary calories and unhealthy fats.

Batch cooking and meal prepping can further simplify the process, allowing for quick access to nutritious meals throughout the week. Having healthy snacks readily available can also help curb cravings and make healthier choices easier.

Lastly, staying hydrated is an often-overlooked aspect of meal planning. Older adults may have a diminished sense of thirst, making it crucial to incorporate fluids into meals. Including soups, smoothies, and water-rich fruits and vegetables can help maintain hydration levels.

Regularly assessing fluid intake and making it a point to drink water throughout the day can aid in digestion and overall health. By adhering to these meal planning tips, older adults can create a framework that supports their journey to prevent frailty and promote strength as they age.

Supplements: Do You Need Them?

Supplements have become a popular topic in discussions about health and wellness, particularly for older adults seeking to prevent frailty. The aging process often leads to changes in nutrient absorption and metabolism, which can make it challenging for individuals to meet their nutritional needs through diet alone.

While a balanced diet rich in whole foods is the cornerstone of good health, some may find it beneficial to consider supplements as an adjunct to their dietary intake. However, understanding whether you need supplements requires careful consideration of various factors, including dietary habits, health status, and lifestyle.

The effectiveness of supplements largely depends on individual nutritional deficiencies and health conditions. For example, older adults may have a higher risk of deficiencies in vitamin D, calcium, and vitamin B12 due to factors such as decreased sun exposure, changes in dietary intake, and reduced absorption in the gastrointestinal tract.

These deficiencies can contribute to muscle weakness, decreased bone density, and an increased risk of falls, all of which are linked to frailty. Conducting a comprehensive assessment of your nutritional status through blood tests and consultations with healthcare professionals can help identify any specific deficiencies and guide supplement use.

It is essential to approach the use of supplements with caution. Not all supplements are created equal, and the market is filled with products that may not be effective or safe. Some supplements can interact with medications, exacerbate existing health conditions, or lead to toxicity if taken in excessive amounts.

Therefore, it is crucial to discuss any potential supplements with a healthcare provider who can provide personalized recommendations based on your health history and current medications. This proactive step can help ensure that any supplements you consider are appropriate and beneficial for your specific situation.

In addition to vitamins and minerals, other supplements such as protein powders, omega-3 fatty acids, and probiotics may also be considered. Protein is vital for maintaining muscle mass, which is essential for preventing frailty. Omega-3 fatty acids have been linked to improved heart health and reduced inflammation, while probiotics can support gut health and enhance nutrient absorption. However, the need for these supplements should still be evaluated on an individual basis, taking into account dietary sources, lifestyle factors, and overall health goals.

Ultimately, while supplements can play a role in supporting health and preventing frailty, they should not replace a well-rounded diet and healthy lifestyle. Prioritizing whole foods, regular physical activity, and proper hydration is fundamental. Supplements can be a useful tool to fill gaps in nutrition, but they should complement rather than substitute for healthy eating habits.

In conclusion, assessing your nutritional needs, consulting with healthcare professionals, and making informed choices about supplements can contribute significantly to your efforts to prevent frailty as you age.

How To Prevent Frailty

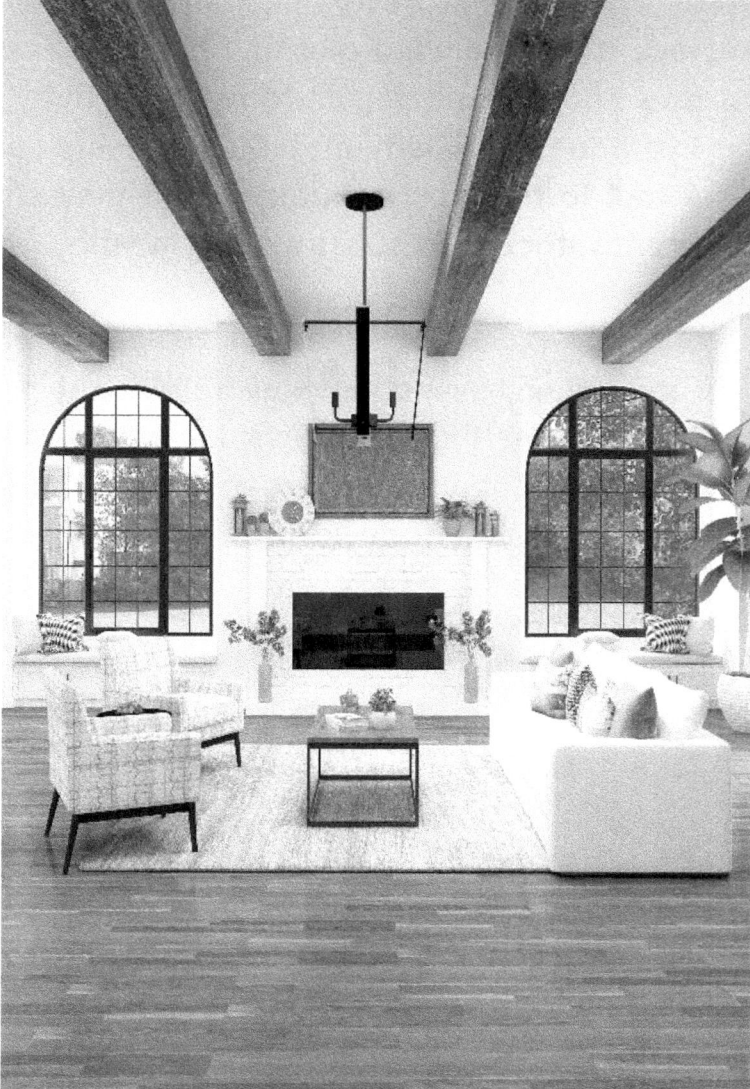

Chapter 4

Creating a Safe Exercise Environment

Assessing Your Home for Safety

Assessing your home for safety is a crucial step in preventing frailty as you age. A safe living environment reduces the risk of falls and accidents, which can lead to significant health challenges. Begin your assessment by walking through each room with a critical eye.

Look for potential hazards such as loose rugs, cluttered walkways, and inadequate lighting. Ensure that pathways are clear and that all areas, especially stairs and hallways, are well-illuminated. Installing brighter bulbs or additional light fixtures may be necessary to enhance visibility.

Next, evaluate the furniture arrangement in your home. Ensure that furniture is placed in a manner that allows for easy navigation without obstacles. Consider the height and stability of furniture, particularly seating options. Chairs should be at an appropriate height to allow for easy sitting and standing.

Be mindful of items that may require bending or stretching to reach, as these movements can increase the risk of falls. Adjusting furniture and storage solutions to create a more accessible environment can significantly contribute to your safety.

Bathroom safety is particularly important, as it is one of the most common places for accidents to occur. Assess the presence of grab bars near the toilet and in the shower or bathtub. Non-slip mats can also reduce the risk of slipping on wet surfaces. Additionally, ensure that the water temperature is regulated to prevent burns.

Consider using a shower chair or a handheld showerhead to make bathing easier and safer. A well-thought-out bathroom can greatly reduce the likelihood of accidents and contribute to your overall well-being.

The kitchen is another area that warrants careful examination. Assess the layout to ensure that frequently used items are within easy reach and do not require excessive bending or stretching. Use non-slip mats in front of the sink and stove to provide stability.

Installing pull-out shelves and using kitchen tools designed for those with limited mobility can also enhance safety. Keeping the kitchen organized and minimizing clutter will help prevent accidents while cooking and preparing meals.

Finally, consider the outdoor spaces surrounding your home. Check for uneven surfaces, such as cracked sidewalks or loose gravel, that could pose a tripping hazard. Ensure that outdoor lighting is adequate for evening use, and remove any debris that may obstruct pathways. Regular maintenance of outdoor areas, including clearing snow or leaves, is essential to prevent slips and falls.

By taking the time to assess and improve the safety of your home, you can create an environment that supports your independence and helps prevent frailty as you age.

Choosing the Right Equipment

Choosing the right equipment is crucial for anyone looking to prevent frailty and maintain strength as they age. The right tools can make a significant difference in not only the effectiveness of workouts but also in ensuring safety and comfort.

When selecting equipment, consider both your current fitness level and your personal goals. Whether you are a beginner or someone with more experience, the equipment should cater to your specific needs while promoting gradual progression.

One of the most versatile pieces of equipment is resistance bands. They are lightweight, portable, and can be used to perform a variety of exercises that target different muscle groups. Resistance bands come in various resistance levels, making them suitable for all fitness levels.

They allow for a full range of motion and can be adjusted to increase or decrease intensity, providing a safe way to build strength without the risk of injury associated with heavier weights.

For those who prefer weight training, dumbbells are an excellent choice. They offer the ability to perform a wide range of exercises and can be easily adjusted to suit individual strength levels. Starting with lighter weights is advisable, allowing for proper form and technique to be established before progressing to heavier loads.

Additionally, adjustable dumbbells can be a space-saving solution, offering various weights in one compact unit. This flexibility makes it easier to incorporate strength training into a regular fitness routine.

Another important consideration is the use of stability balls or balance boards. These tools not only aid in strength training but also improve balance and core stability, which are critical components in preventing falls and injuries. Incorporating exercises that engage the core while using these tools can enhance overall body strength and coordination.

Furthermore, they encourage proper posture and alignment, which is essential as one ages, helping to mitigate the risk of frailty.

Finally, it is essential to prioritize safety when selecting any fitness equipment. Look for items that have a good reputation for durability and user-friendliness. Equipment should be stable and easy to handle, ensuring that workouts can be performed without fear of accidents.

Additionally, consider consulting with a fitness professional when making your selections, as they can provide valuable insights and recommendations tailored to your individual needs. By choosing the right equipment, you set a solid foundation for a successful strength-building regimen that will help you prevent frailty and enhance your quality of life as you age.

Finding the Right Space for Exercise

Finding the right space for exercise is crucial for anyone aiming to prevent frailty as they age. The environment in which you choose to work out can significantly influence your motivation, safety, and overall enjoyment of physical activity. Whether you prefer exercising at home, in a gym, or outdoors, it is essential to consider several factors that will contribute to a positive experience.

When selecting a home space for exercise, consider the size and layout of the area. A dedicated room or a corner of your living space can be ideal for setting up workout equipment and creating an inviting atmosphere.

Make sure the area is free from clutter and hazards to prevent injuries. Good lighting is also important, as it can enhance your mood and energy levels during workouts. If you have limited space, consider multipurpose equipment that can be easily stored away when not in use.

For those who prefer a gym environment, choosing the right facility is key. Look for gyms that cater to your specific fitness level and goals. Many gyms offer specialized programs for older adults, with trainers skilled in working with individuals looking to maintain strength and mobility.

Assess the gym's equipment availability, cleanliness, and overall atmosphere. A welcoming environment with supportive staff can make a significant difference in your commitment to regular exercise.

Outdoor spaces can provide a refreshing alternative to indoor workouts. Parks, nature trails, and community spaces offer ample opportunities for walking, jogging, or group classes. Consider the accessibility of these locations and whether they are safe and comfortable for your fitness routine. Exercising outdoors can also boost mental health and provide a sense of community, as you may encounter others who share your fitness goals.

Finally, it is important to personalize your exercise space based on your preferences and needs. Incorporate elements that inspire you, such as motivational quotes, music, or visual reminders of your fitness goals.

If you enjoy social interaction, consider inviting friends or family to join you in your exercise routine. A supportive network can enhance your commitment to staying active and help you find joy in the process, ultimately contributing to the prevention of frailty as you age.

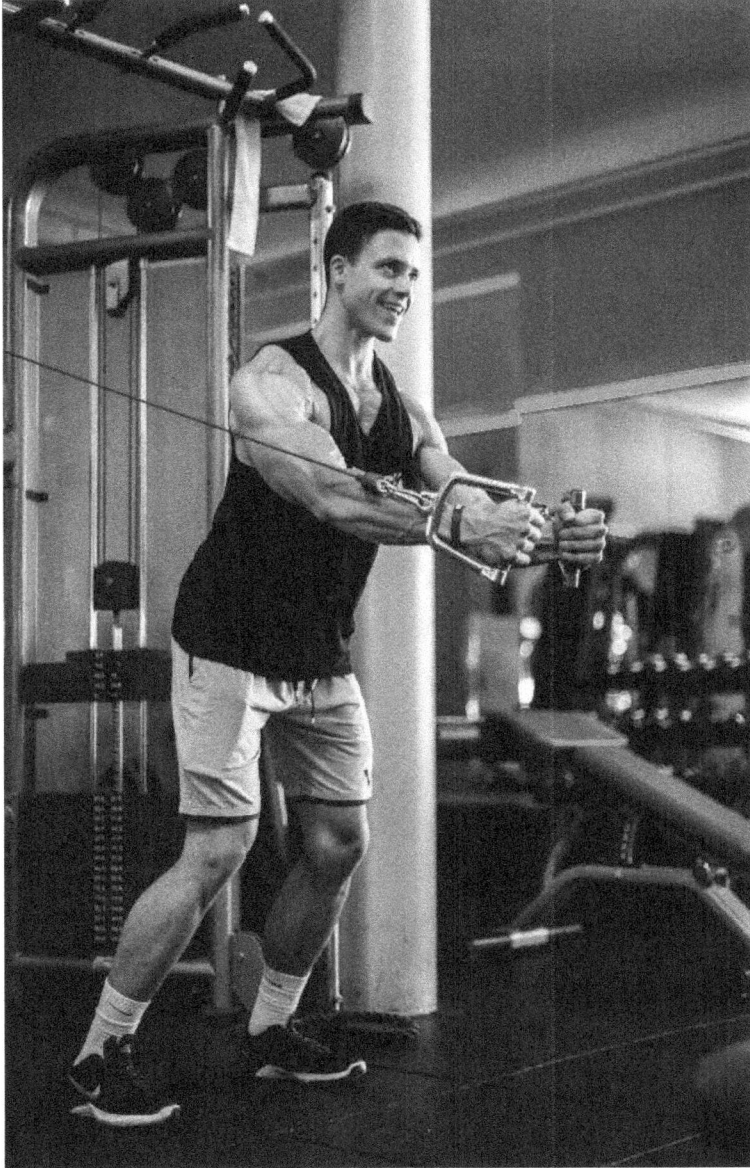

Chapter 5

Developing a Personalized Strength Training Program

Assessing Your Current Fitness Level

Assessing your current fitness level is a critical first step in preventing frailty as you age. Understanding where you stand in terms of physical health can help you identify areas that need improvement and set realistic goals for your fitness journey.

To effectively assess your fitness level, consider evaluating various components such as aerobic capacity, muscular strength, endurance, flexibility, and balance. Each of these factors plays a vital role in maintaining overall health and functionality as you grow older.

One effective way to gauge your aerobic capacity is through a simple walking test. Begin with a brisk walk for six minutes, then measure the distance covered. This distance can provide insights into your cardiovascular fitness.

If you're unable to walk for an extended period, consider alternative activities like cycling or swimming, which can also help assess your stamina. Documenting your heart rate before and after the activity can further enhance your understanding of your aerobic endurance and recovery capability.

Muscular strength can be assessed through various exercises that target major muscle groups. The chair stand test is a practical and effective method for older adults. It involves sitting in a sturdy chair and standing up as many times as possible within 30 seconds.

The number of repetitions completed indicates your lower body strength, which is crucial for daily activities and overall mobility. Additionally, incorporating push-ups or wall push-ups can help you evaluate upper body strength, another essential component of fitness.

Flexibility is often overlooked but is equally important in preventing frailty. Simple stretching exercises can help you assess your range of motion. The sit-and-reach test is a common method where you sit on the floor with your legs extended and reach towards your toes. Measuring how far you can reach provides a clear picture of your flexibility. Regular flexibility assessments can help prevent injuries and improve your ability to perform everyday tasks, enhancing your overall quality of life.

Balance is a critical aspect of fitness, particularly as you age, due to its direct correlation with fall prevention. The single-leg stand test is a straightforward way to assess your balance. Stand on one leg while keeping the other raised, and time how long you can maintain that position without support.

A longer duration indicates better balance, which is essential for stability and independence. Regularly assessing these fitness components will not only help you track your progress but also empower you to make informed decisions about your exercise regimen, ultimately aiding in the prevention of frailty.

Setting Realistic Goals

Setting realistic goals is a fundamental step in any journey toward preventing frailty and maintaining strength as one ages. Realistic goals serve as a roadmap, providing direction and motivation while ensuring that individuals stay committed to their health and wellness.

When goals are attainable, they help foster a sense of accomplishment, which can be particularly important for older adults who may have experienced challenges in their physical health or mobility. By carefully considering the nature of these goals, individuals can create a sustainable plan that encourages consistent effort and progress.

To begin setting realistic goals, it is essential to conduct a self-assessment. This involves evaluating current physical abilities, health status, and lifestyle habits. Understanding where one stands allows for the establishment of clear and achievable targets. For example, if the goal is to increase physical activity, it is vital to consider current activity levels and any limitations.

Aiming to walk for 30 minutes a day may be unrealistic for someone who is currently sedentary. Instead, starting with 10-minute walks and gradually increasing duration can lead to better adherence and overall improvement.

Another critical aspect of goal setting is the SMART criteria: Specific, Measurable, Achievable, Relevant, and Time-bound. Each goal should clearly outline what is to be accomplished, how success will be measured, and the timeframe for completion.

For instance, instead of a vague goal like "I want to be stronger," a SMART goal would be "I will perform two strength training sessions each week for the next three months." This approach not only clarifies the goal but also makes it easier to track progress and make adjustments as needed.

It is also important to recognize that setbacks and challenges are a natural part of the process. Aging often brings unexpected health issues, changes in energy levels, or other unforeseen circumstances that can hinder progress.

Embracing a flexible mindset and adjusting goals as needed can help maintain motivation and prevent discouragement. For example, if a planned exercise routine becomes too strenuous, modifying the frequency or intensity of workouts can lead to continued engagement without risking injury or burnout.

Lastly, celebrating small victories is essential for maintaining motivation along the way. Acknowledging progress, no matter how minor it may seem, can reinforce the commitment to the overall goal. Whether it is completing an exercise session or achieving a personal best in strength, recognizing these moments encourages further effort and builds confidence.

Setting realistic goals, adjusting them as necessary, and celebrating achievements together create a holistic approach to preventing frailty and enhancing overall well-being as one ages.

Types of Strength Training Exercises

Strength training exercises can be categorized into several types, each offering unique benefits that contribute to overall strength, balance, and functionality. Understanding these types is crucial for individuals looking to prevent frailty as they age.

The primary categories include bodyweight exercises, free weights, resistance machines, resistance bands, and functional training exercises. Each type plays a distinct role in enhancing muscle strength and endurance, which are vital in maintaining independence and mobility in later years.

Bodyweight exercises utilize the individual's own weight as resistance. These exercises, such as push-ups, squats, and lunges, can be performed anywhere and require no special equipment. They are particularly beneficial for beginners as they focus on mastering form and technique before progressing to more advanced movements. Additionally, bodyweight exercises can be easily modified to suit varying fitness levels, making them accessible for older adults who may be just starting their strength training journey.

Free weights, including dumbbells and kettlebells, are another effective type of strength training. These weights allow for a range of motion and can target specific muscle groups, promoting balanced muscle development. Free weight exercises such as bicep curls, shoulder presses, and deadlifts enhance both strength and coordination.

For those concerned about safety, starting with lighter weights and gradually increasing resistance can help individuals build confidence and avoid injury.

Resistance machines are often found in gyms and fitness centers, designed to provide a controlled environment for strength training. These machines isolate specific muscle groups, making it easier for users to focus on particular areas of strength without the need for a spotter.

While they can be beneficial for beginners, it's important to learn proper usage to avoid strain or injury. Machines can be particularly useful for older adults as they often provide adjustable settings to accommodate varying levels of strength and mobility.

Resistance bands are a versatile and portable option for strength training. They come in different resistance levels, allowing users to adjust the intensity of their workouts easily. Resistance bands are effective for both upper and lower body exercises, such as banded squats or seated rows.

They also promote joint stability and can be particularly beneficial for rehabilitation purposes. Finally, functional training exercises mimic everyday movements, enhancing balance and coordination. Exercises like step-ups, kettlebell swings, and medicine ball throws help improve the ability to perform daily activities with ease, ultimately reducing the risk of falls and injuries as one ages.

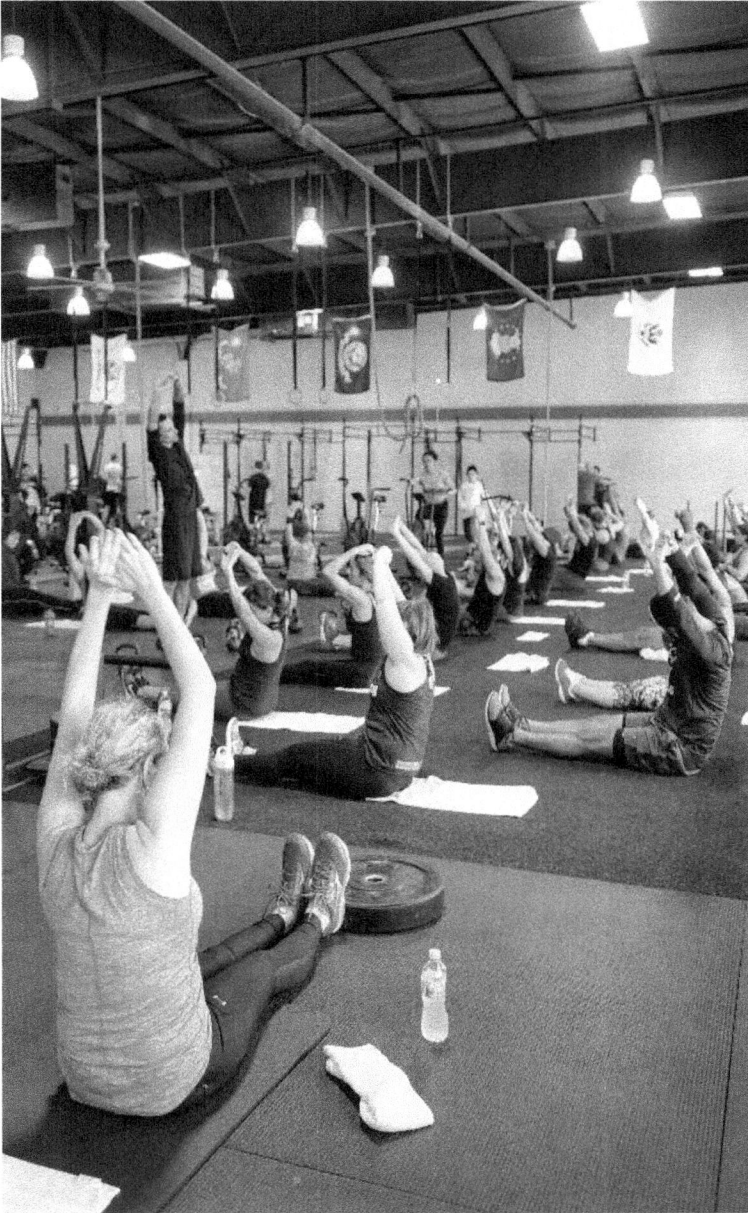

Chapter 6

Incorporating Flexibility and Balance Training

The Role of Flexibility in Preventing Frailty

Flexibility plays a crucial role in preventing frailty as individuals age. As the body ages, muscles and joints naturally lose some of their elasticity and range of motion. This decline can lead to stiffness and discomfort, which may discourage physical activity.

By maintaining and enhancing flexibility through regular stretching and mobility exercises, individuals can preserve their physical capabilities, reduce the risk of injury, and improve overall functional performance. Engaging in flexibility training helps to counteract the natural aging process, allowing older adults to remain more active and independent.

Incorporating flexibility exercises into a routine can significantly influence balance and coordination. As flexibility improves, it also enhances the body's ability to move smoothly and efficiently. This is particularly important for older adults who may already be at risk of falls due to decreased balance and coordination.

By enhancing flexibility, individuals can better control their movements and react quickly to prevent falls. Simple activities such as yoga or tai chi not only promote flexibility but also focus on balance, making them ideal for frailty prevention.

Moreover, flexibility exercises can alleviate muscle tension and soreness, which are common complaints among older adults. This reduction in discomfort can lead to a more active lifestyle, encouraging individuals to engage in physical activities that they may have previously avoided due to pain or stiffness.

Regularly stretching major muscle groups not only enhances flexibility but also promotes blood circulation, which is beneficial for overall muscle health. As older adults experience less discomfort, they are more likely to participate in exercise programs that build strength and endurance, further combating the onset of frailty.

Mental well-being is another significant aspect of flexibility training that should not be overlooked. Engaging in flexibility exercises can have a meditative effect, reducing stress and anxiety levels. This mental clarity can motivate individuals to maintain their physical health and wellness routines.

A positive mindset can help foster a sense of achievement and encourage ongoing participation in physical activity, which is essential for preventing frailty. By prioritizing flexibility, individuals can create a holistic approach to their health that encompasses both physical and mental resilience.

Lastly, flexibility training can be easily integrated into daily routines, making it accessible for individuals of varying fitness levels. Whether through dedicated stretching sessions, incorporating flexibility into warm-up and cool-down periods of exercise, or participating in group classes, there are numerous ways to enhance flexibility.

Simple stretches can be performed at home without the need for special equipment, making it a convenient option. By adopting a flexible routine, older adults can empower themselves to take charge of their health and work proactively toward preventing frailty as they age.

Balance Exercises to Reduce Fall Risk

Balance exercises play a crucial role in reducing fall risk, especially as individuals age and become more susceptible to frailty. Maintaining good balance is essential for everyday activities, and engaging in targeted exercises can significantly enhance stability and coordination.

These exercises not only improve physical strength but also foster confidence, allowing individuals to navigate their environments with greater assurance. Understanding the importance of balance training is the first step toward preventing falls and promoting overall well-being.

One effective approach to balance training involves incorporating simple exercises into daily routines. Activities such as standing on one leg, heel-to-toe walking, and practicing gentle yoga poses can enhance balance and stability.

These exercises can be performed in the comfort of one's home and require minimal equipment, making them accessible to a wide range of individuals. Starting with basic movements and gradually increasing difficulty can help build strength and proprioception, which is the body's ability to sense its position in space.

In addition to individual exercises, incorporating balance-enhancing activities into social or group settings can be particularly beneficial. Classes focused on tai chi or dance not only provide structured environments for practicing balance but also foster social connections, which are vital for mental health and motivation.

Participating in group exercises can create a sense of accountability and encourage consistency, ultimately leading to better outcomes in terms of fall prevention and overall fitness.

It is also important to consider the environment when engaging in balance exercises. Creating a safe space free from potential hazards, such as loose rugs or clutter, can significantly reduce the risk of falls during practice. Using supportive equipment, such as sturdy chairs or wall bars for assistance, can provide additional safety while individuals work on their balance skills.

Ensuring that exercise areas are well-lit and free from obstacles will help participants focus on their movements without the distraction of environmental risks.

Regularly incorporating balance exercises into a fitness routine can lead to long-term benefits beyond just fall prevention. Improved balance can enhance overall mobility, increase independence, and contribute to better quality of life as individuals age. By prioritizing balance training and making it a consistent part of daily life, individuals can take proactive steps toward reducing their risk of falls, thereby combating frailty and promoting a healthier, more active lifestyle.

Combining Flexibility and Strength Training

Combining flexibility and strength training is essential for preventing frailty as we age. Flexibility exercises enhance the range of motion in joints, which is crucial for maintaining mobility and preventing injuries. As we grow older, our muscles and connective tissues naturally lose elasticity, making it imperative to incorporate flexibility routines into our fitness regimen.

Stretching not only improves flexibility but also promotes circulation and reduces muscle soreness, allowing for more effective strength training sessions.

Strength training is equally important in the fight against frailty. It involves exercises that improve muscle strength, endurance, and overall stability. Engaging in regular strength training helps to build and maintain muscle mass, which tends to decline with age. This decline can lead to weakness and increased risk of falls.

By incorporating resistance exercises, whether through weights, resistance bands, or bodyweight movements, individuals can enhance their muscle strength and support their skeletal structure, leading to improved balance and functional mobility.

The synergy between flexibility and strength training is particularly beneficial. When strength training is paired with flexibility exercises, individuals can achieve better overall physical performance. For example, a strong muscle is more effective when it can move freely through its full range of motion. Flexibility allows for greater strength output and reduces the risk of injury during strength training routines. Therefore, a well-rounded exercise program should integrate both aspects for optimal results.

In practice, combining these two elements can take various forms. A balanced workout might begin with dynamic stretches to warm up the body, followed by strength training exercises targeting major muscle groups. After the strength component, static stretching can be employed to cool down and improve flexibility. This structure not only promotes physical health but also encourages mindfulness and body awareness, further supporting the prevention of frailty.

Ultimately, the integration of flexibility and strength training holds the key to maintaining functional independence as we age. Individuals who prioritize both components will likely experience enhanced physical capabilities, reduced injury risk, and improved quality of life. By understanding the importance of this combination and committing to a comprehensive fitness routine, one can effectively combat the effects of aging and stave off frailty.

How To Prevent Frailty

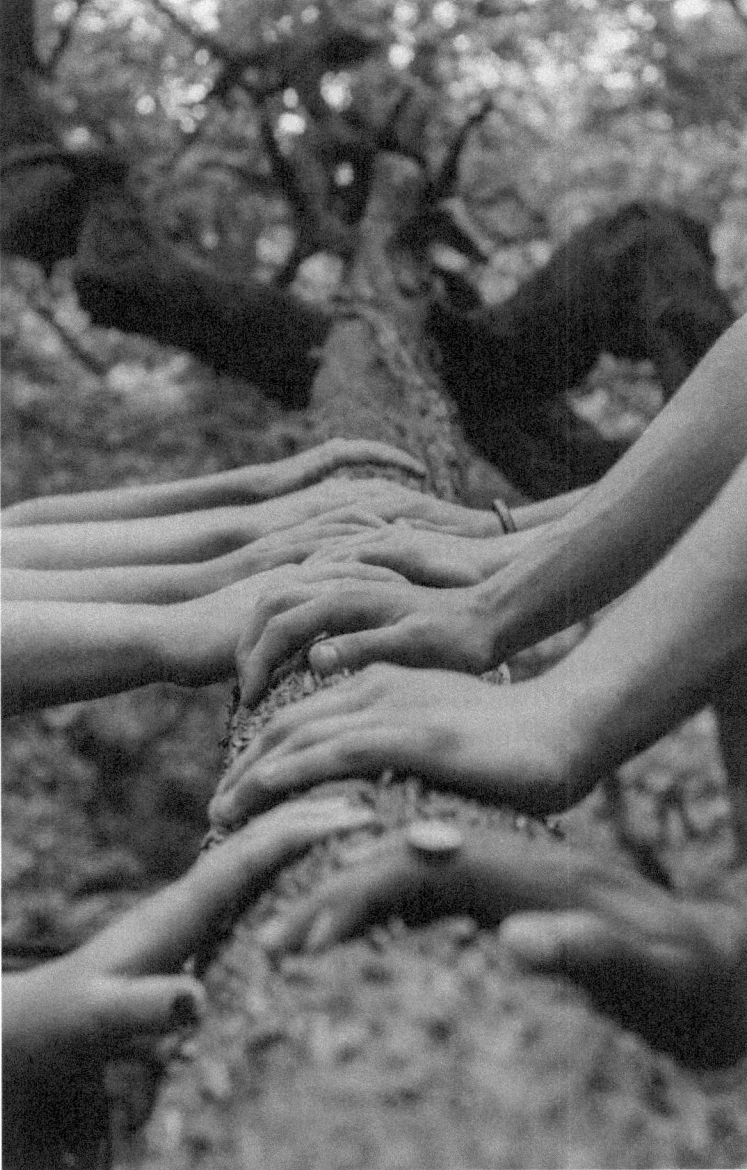

Chapter 7

The Role of Social Connections

Building a Support Network

Building a strong support network is crucial for individuals aiming to prevent frailty as they age. A support network can consist of family, friends, neighbors, and community resources that provide emotional, social, and practical assistance.

Engaging with a variety of people can not only enhance one's sense of belonging but also serve as a buffer against the challenges associated with aging. The interactions within this network can contribute to mental well-being, which is integral to maintaining physical health and resilience.

One of the first steps in establishing a support network is to identify individuals who can play a role in this system. Family members often take on this role naturally, but it is essential to recognize that friends and acquaintances can also provide significant support.

It may be beneficial to reach out to neighbors or join local clubs and organizations that align with personal interests. This approach not only expands social circles but also facilitates connections with like-minded individuals who share similar goals related to health and well-being.

In addition to personal relationships, professional resources can enhance a support network. Healthcare providers, such as primary care physicians, physical therapists, and nutritionists, can offer expert guidance on maintaining strength and preventing frailty. Community centers and local health organizations may also provide classes, workshops, or group activities focused on fitness, nutrition, and mental health. Connecting with these professionals can equip individuals with valuable information and skills that contribute to overall wellness.

Engaging with support networks requires active participation. Regularly attending social gatherings, participating in group activities, or even volunteering can foster stronger relationships and create a sense of purpose. Encouraging open communication within the network can lead to better understanding and increased support. Additionally, sharing personal experiences and challenges can inspire others to contribute or provide assistance, thereby reinforcing the network's strength and resilience.

Finally, it is essential to maintain and nurture these connections over time. Regular check-ins with network members, whether through phone calls, messages, or in-person visits, can help sustain relationships and ensure ongoing support.

As life circumstances change—such as moving to a new location or experiencing health changes—adapting the support network is vital. By continuously building and maintaining a diverse support network, individuals can foster an environment that promotes strength, resilience, and a higher quality of life as they age.

Group Activities and Classes

Engaging in group activities and classes is an effective strategy for preventing frailty as individuals age. These social and physical engagements not only foster a sense of community but also provide opportunities for regular exercise, which is crucial for maintaining strength and mobility. Participating in group activities can encourage individuals to push themselves further than they might when exercising alone, leading to improved physical fitness and a reduced risk of frailty.

Fitness classes specifically designed for older adults can be especially beneficial. These classes often focus on low-impact exercises that enhance strength, balance, and flexibility, all of which are essential for daily functioning and injury prevention.

Activities such as yoga, tai chi, and water aerobics are popular options that help to build core strength while also promoting relaxation and mental well-being. Additionally, these classes are typically led by trained instructors who understand the unique needs of older adults, ensuring a safe and supportive environment.

Beyond physical benefits, group activities provide significant social advantages. Loneliness and isolation can contribute to the decline in physical and mental health, making social connections critical as we age. Group classes create a space where individuals can meet others with similar interests, fostering friendships and enhancing social networks.

This interaction can lead to increased motivation to attend classes regularly, creating a positive feedback loop that reinforces both social engagement and physical activity.

Incorporating various group activities into one's routine can also keep the experience fresh and exciting. This could include joining a dance class, participating in community gardening, or engaging in group walks or hikes.

The diversity of activities available allows individuals to find something they genuinely enjoy, which is vital for long-term adherence to an active lifestyle. Experimenting with different classes can also help uncover new interests, making exercise a more enjoyable and fulfilling part of daily life.

To maximize the benefits of group activities and classes, it is important to approach these opportunities with an open mind and a willingness to participate fully. Setting personal goals, such as attending a certain number of classes each week or trying a new activity each month, can further enhance the experience.

By committing to a routine that includes group activities, individuals not only work towards preventing frailty but also enrich their lives through social connections and shared experiences.

The Psychological Benefits of Social Interaction

Social interaction plays a crucial role in mental and emotional well-being, particularly as individuals age. Engaging with others not only fosters a sense of belonging but also helps to alleviate feelings of loneliness and isolation.

Studies have consistently shown that individuals who maintain regular social interactions tend to experience lower levels of anxiety and depression. The simple act of conversing with friends, family, or community members can serve as a protective factor against the cognitive decline often associated with aging.

This interaction stimulates the brain, encouraging the formation of new neural connections and enhancing overall cognitive function.

The benefits of social interaction extend beyond emotional health; they also significantly impact physical health. Research indicates that individuals who engage socially are more likely to adopt healthier lifestyles. This includes regular physical activity, better dietary choices, and adherence to medical advice.

Social connections can motivate individuals to participate in group exercises or wellness activities, creating a supportive environment that encourages healthier habits. As a result, these positive lifestyle choices contribute to improved physical strength and resilience, which are essential in preventing frailty.

Moreover, social interaction can increase longevity. A wealth of research suggests that strong social ties correlate with a longer lifespan. Individuals who cultivate and maintain relationships tend to have lower stress levels, which is a significant factor in overall health.

Chronic stress can lead to various health issues, including heart disease and weakened immune response. By fostering connections and engaging in meaningful conversations, individuals can reduce stress and promote a sense of happiness and fulfillment, ultimately contributing to a longer, healthier life.

Additionally, social engagement provides opportunities for learning and intellectual stimulation. Participating in group activities, attending workshops, or simply sharing experiences with others can enhance cognitive function and memory retention. This intellectual engagement keeps the mind sharp and active, which is vital in combating cognitive decline. Lifelong learning through social interaction encourages curiosity and creativity, allowing individuals to continue growing and adapting throughout their lives.

Lastly, the sense of community created through social interaction can enhance one's sense of purpose. Feeling connected to others and contributing to the well-being of friends or community members fosters a feeling of significance and fulfillment.

This sense of purpose is crucial in combating the feelings of worthlessness or despair that can accompany aging. As individuals engage with their communities and support one another, they not only enhance their own lives but also create a positive ripple effect that strengthens the social fabric of their environments.

By recognizing the psychological benefits of social interaction, individuals can take proactive steps to foster connections that enrich their lives and help prevent frailty as they age.

How To Prevent Frailty

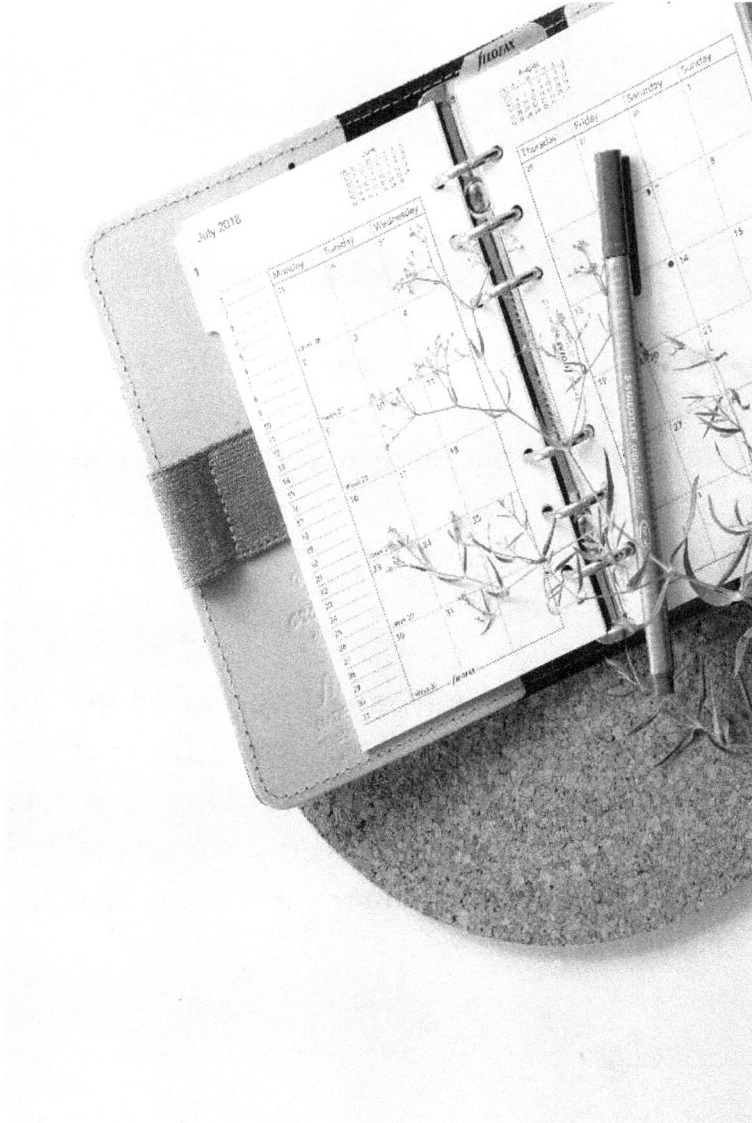

Chapter 8

Monitoring Progress and Staying Motivated

Tracking Your Strength Gains

Tracking your strength gains is a crucial component in the journey to prevent frailty as you age. By systematically recording your progress, you not only gain insight into your physical capabilities but also enhance your motivation to continue your strength training regimen.

This practice involves noting the exercises you perform, the weights used, and the number of repetitions or sets completed. Over time, this data will provide a clear picture of your improvements, helping you to identify trends and make informed adjustments to your training routine.

One effective method for tracking your strength gains is to maintain a workout log. This log can be a simple notebook or a digital app where you record each session's details. Including the date, exercises performed, weights lifted, and your perceived level of effort will allow you to visualize changes in performance.

By regularly reviewing this log, you can celebrate small victories and set realistic goals. For instance, if you notice that you are able to lift more weight or complete additional repetitions, it serves as a tangible reminder of your hard work and commitment.

In addition to quantitative measures, qualitative assessments can enrich your tracking process. Pay attention to how you feel during and after workouts. Are you experiencing less fatigue than when you started? Do your movements feel more fluid and less strained?

These subjective indicators are just as important as numerical data. They can help you gauge your overall well-being and physical condition, providing a more comprehensive understanding of your strength gains.

Incorporating regular assessments is another way to track progress effectively. Consider scheduling monthly evaluations where you perform a set of standard exercises to measure your strength. This could include squats, deadlifts, or push-ups, using consistent weights and repetitions each time.

Documenting these assessments will highlight improvements in your performance and can be a motivating factor to continue pushing your limits. It also allows you to adjust your training program to ensure ongoing challenges to your muscles, preventing plateaus in your strength development.

Lastly, sharing your progress with a coach or a workout partner can further enhance your tracking efforts. They can provide valuable feedback, accountability, and encouragement. Discussing your goals and achievements with someone else not only keeps you motivated but can also introduce new strategies to your training.

This social aspect of tracking strength gains can make the process more enjoyable and sustainable, ultimately contributing to your success in preventing frailty as you age.

Adjusting Your Program as You Progress

As you embark on your journey to prevent frailty, it is essential to recognize that your fitness program should be dynamic rather than static. Adjusting your program as you progress is crucial to continue building strength and endurance while catering to your evolving needs.

This adaptability will help you maintain motivation, avoid plateaus, and ensure that your routine remains aligned with your health and fitness goals. Regular assessments of your progress can provide valuable insights into when and how to make these adjustments.

One of the first indicators that it might be time to adjust your program is your current fitness level. As you become stronger and more capable, the exercises that once challenged you may no longer provide the same level of difficulty. This may necessitate an increase in the intensity of your workouts, whether through higher weights, more challenging variations of exercises, or increased repetitions.

Gradually elevating the difficulty ensures that your muscles continue to be stimulated, promoting growth and strength development.

Another important factor to consider is how your body responds to your current program. Pay attention to signs of fatigue, soreness, or even pain. While some discomfort is normal when exercising, persistent or sharp pain can indicate that your body needs a break or a modification in your routine.

Incorporating rest days, varying your workout types, or switching to lower-impact exercises can help mitigate these issues. Listening to your body is crucial for long-term success, as it allows you to adapt your program to prevent injuries and promote recovery.

In addition to listening to your body, it is beneficial to reassess your goals periodically. As you progress, your objectives may change. Initially, you might focus on building foundational strength, but as you become more confident, you may wish to set new goals such as improving balance, increasing flexibility, or enhancing cardiovascular endurance.

Adjusting your program to align with these shifting goals can keep you engaged and motivated, ensuring that you are continually working toward something that excites you.

Finally, consider incorporating variety into your program to prevent boredom and maintain engagement. This could involve trying new classes, incorporating different types of resistance training, or even exploring outdoor activities.

Variety not only keeps your workouts fun but also challenges your body in new ways, which can lead to improved strength and overall fitness. By adjusting your program as you progress, you create a sustainable routine that not only helps prevent frailty but also enhances your quality of life as you age.

Celebrating Milestones

Celebrating milestones in the journey of aging and health can significantly enhance motivation and reinforce positive behaviors. As individuals strive to prevent frailty, recognizing achievements—whether large or small—can serve as a powerful reminder of their progress.

Milestones can encompass a range of achievements, from completing a specific exercise program to reaching a personal health target, such as improved flexibility or stamina. By acknowledging these accomplishments, individuals can foster a sense of purpose and encourage continued dedication to their health routines.

One effective way to celebrate milestones is to set specific, measurable goals. These goals should be realistic and attainable, allowing individuals to experience success along the way. For instance, someone aiming to increase their strength might set a goal of being able to perform a certain number of bodyweight squats or lift a specified weight.

Tracking progress toward these goals provides tangible evidence of improvement and creates opportunities for celebration when targets are met. This process not only boosts confidence but also reinforces the positive behaviors that contribute to a healthier, more active lifestyle.

Sharing achievements with friends, family, or a supportive community can amplify the celebration of milestones. When individuals share their successes, they invite encouragement and recognition from others, which can reinforce their commitment to ongoing health efforts. Social connections play a critical role in maintaining motivation, as positive reinforcement from peers can lead to greater accountability and adherence to health practices.

Participating in group activities or challenges can also create a sense of camaraderie, where individuals collectively celebrate each other's milestones and support one another in their journeys.

Incorporating rituals or personal rewards can enhance the significance of milestones. For example, treating oneself to a favorite healthy meal, enjoying a relaxing day out, or participating in a fun activity can serve as a reward for achieving health-related goals. These rewards should align with the overall objective of maintaining or improving health, ensuring that they contribute positively to the individual's well-being.

Establishing a routine that includes these celebrations can create a positive feedback loop, encouraging individuals to continue setting and achieving new goals.

Ultimately, celebrating milestones is a vital component of preventing frailty and promoting a strong, healthy lifestyle as one ages. By recognizing and honoring progress, individuals can maintain motivation, strengthen their resolve, and cultivate a positive relationship with their health journey.

As they celebrate each step forward, they not only enhance their physical well-being but also enrich their emotional and social lives, paving the way for a fulfilling, active, and resilient aging experience.

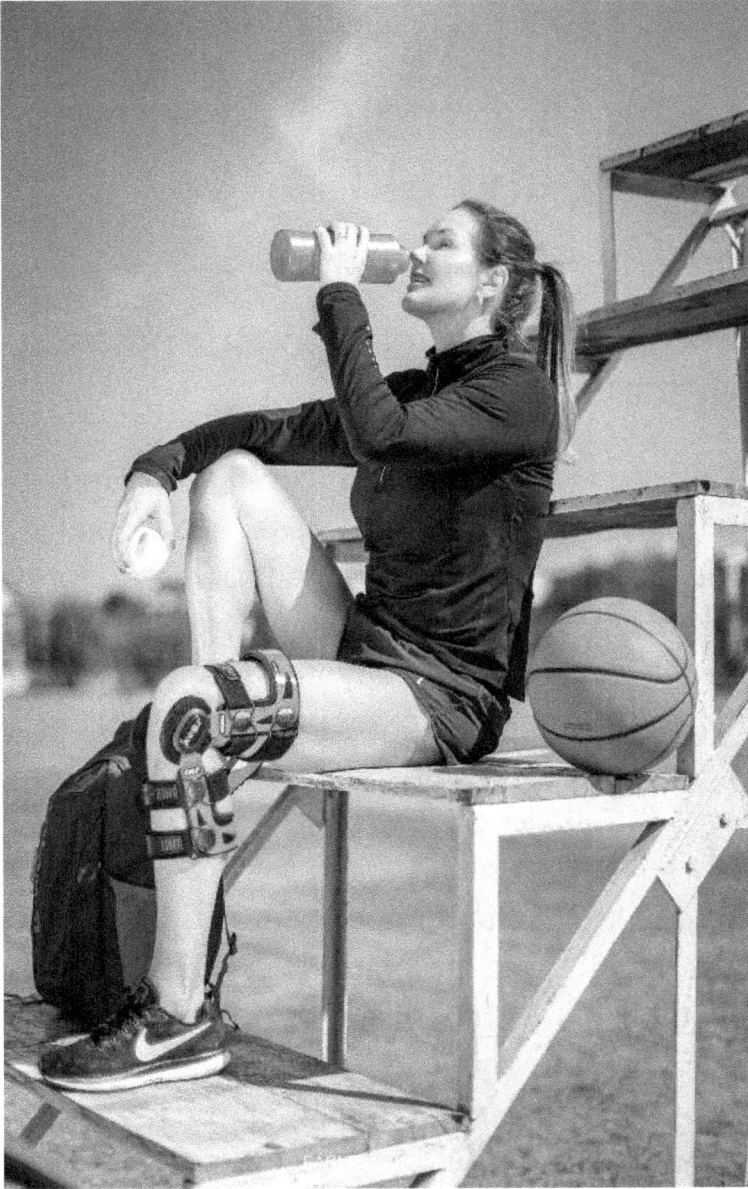

Chapter 9

Overcoming Challenges and Setbacks

Common Obstacles to Strength Training

Common obstacles to strength training can significantly impede progress, especially for individuals aiming to prevent frailty. One major hurdle is the misconception that strength training is only for the young or those already fit. Many older adults believe that engaging in resistance exercises could lead to injury or exacerbate existing health issues.

This belief often stems from a lack of understanding about appropriate modifications and the benefits of strength training for maintaining muscle mass, enhancing balance, and improving overall health. Education about the safety and advantages of strength training can help dispel these myths and encourage participation.

Another common obstacle is physical limitations or chronic health conditions. Many individuals may be dealing with arthritis, osteoporosis, or cardiovascular issues that make traditional strength training routines seem daunting. These concerns can lead to a reluctance to begin or maintain a strength training regimen.

However, there are numerous adaptive exercises and low-impact options available that can accommodate various physical abilities. Consulting with a healthcare professional or a certified trainer who specializes in working with older adults can help develop a customized plan that considers individual limitations while still promoting strength gains.

Motivation plays a crucial role in the success of any fitness program, and a lack of motivation can be a significant barrier to consistent strength training. Older adults may feel discouraged by slow progress or may not see immediate results, leading to frustration and a decrease in adherence to their training routine.

Setting realistic goals and celebrating small achievements can help maintain motivation. Joining a group class or finding a workout partner can also provide social support and accountability, making the process more enjoyable and less isolating.

Time constraints often serve as an obstacle as well. Many individuals lead busy lives, juggling family responsibilities, work, and other commitments, leaving little time for exercise. This can lead to the perception that strength training requires a significant time investment. However, effective strength training does not necessarily require long sessions.

Short, focused workouts can be just as beneficial and can be easily integrated into a busy schedule. Planning a routine that includes two to three sessions a week for 20 to 30 minutes can yield substantial benefits without overwhelming time commitments.

Lastly, access to facilities and equipment can pose challenges for those looking to engage in strength training. Not everyone has a gym membership or the means to purchase equipment for home use. This concern can deter individuals from even starting a strength training program.

Fortunately, many bodyweight exercises require no equipment and can be performed anywhere. Additionally, community centers, local gyms, or senior centers often offer affordable classes that focus on strength training. Exploring these options can provide the necessary resources to overcome financial or logistical barriers, enabling individuals to prioritize their strength training efforts as part of their frailty prevention strategy.

Strategies for Staying on Track

Staying on track with health and wellness goals is essential for preventing frailty as you age. One of the most effective strategies is to establish a routine that incorporates physical activity, balanced nutrition, and mental engagement.

Creating a daily schedule that includes specific times for exercise, meal preparation, and social activities can make it easier to adhere to these practices. Consistency is key; by integrating healthy habits into your daily life, you build a strong foundation that supports your overall well-being.

Setting realistic and achievable goals is another important strategy. It is crucial to break larger objectives into smaller, manageable steps. For instance, if the aim is to engage in regular exercise, start with short sessions of walking or low-impact activities and gradually increase the duration and intensity. Keeping track of your progress can be motivating and help you identify any obstacles you may encounter. Use tools like journals or apps to record your achievements, which can serve as a source of encouragement and accountability.

Social support plays a vital role in maintaining motivation and staying on track. Engaging with friends, family, or community groups can provide a sense of belonging and accountability. Consider participating in group exercise classes, cooking sessions, or community events focused on wellness.

Sharing your goals with others can also lead to mutual encouragement, and you may find that someone else is on a similar journey. Social interactions not only enhance motivation but also contribute to emotional well-being, which is crucial in preventing frailty.

Incorporating variety into your routine can prevent boredom and burnout. Explore different types of physical activity, such as swimming, dancing, or yoga, to keep your workouts interesting. Experiment with new healthy recipes to maintain a balanced diet, ensuring your meals remain appealing and nutritious.

This variety can stimulate both your body and mind, making it easier to stay committed to your health goals. Additionally, learning new skills or hobbies can provide mental stimulation, further supporting your overall health.

Finally, it is essential to practice self-compassion and flexibility. Life can be unpredictable, and setbacks may occur. Instead of being overly critical of yourself when things don't go as planned, approach challenges with a positive mindset.

Allow yourself the grace to adapt your goals as necessary and recognize that maintaining your health is a lifelong journey. By fostering a compassionate attitude toward yourself, you can sustain motivation and resilience, crucial components in your quest to prevent frailty as you age.

Dealing with Injuries and Recovery

Dealing with injuries and recovery is a critical aspect of maintaining strength and preventing frailty as we age. Injuries can occur unexpectedly, whether from a fall, overexertion, or an underlying health condition.

Understanding the common types of injuries that affect older adults, as well as the importance of timely and appropriate recovery strategies, can significantly impact overall health and well-being. Acknowledging the reality of injuries allows individuals to adopt proactive measures that can facilitate quicker recovery and support long-term strength.

One of the most prevalent injuries among older adults is a fall, which can lead to fractures, sprains, or other musculoskeletal injuries. Falls often result from factors such as decreased balance, muscle weakness, or environmental hazards. To prevent such injuries, it is crucial to engage in regular balance and strength training exercises that enhance stability.

Additionally, creating a safe living environment by removing tripping hazards and ensuring adequate lighting can further mitigate the risk of falls. By adopting these preventive strategies, individuals can reduce the likelihood of injuries that may hinder their ability to maintain strength and independence.

In the event of an injury, a prompt response is essential for effective recovery. Initial treatment often involves rest, ice, compression, and elevation, commonly referred to as the RICE method. Following this, seeking medical advice for a tailored rehabilitation plan can ensure that recovery is both safe and effective.

Rehabilitation may include physical therapy, which focuses on restoring mobility, strength, and function. Engaging with a qualified professional can provide personalized guidance, helping individuals safely navigate their recovery process and avoid setbacks that could lead to prolonged frailty.

Mental and emotional well-being also plays a significant role in recovery from injuries. The psychological impact of an injury can lead to feelings of frustration, anxiety, or depression, which may hinder motivation to engage in rehabilitation activities. It is important to cultivate a positive mindset and maintain social connections during the recovery phase.

Encouragement from family, friends, or support groups can foster resilience and promote adherence to recovery plans. Practicing mindfulness or engaging in enjoyable activities can also help manage stress and improve overall emotional health during this challenging time.

Ultimately, dealing with injuries and recovery is an integral part of a holistic approach to preventing frailty. By prioritizing injury prevention, responding effectively to injuries when they occur, and nurturing mental well-being, older adults can maintain their strength and independence. Emphasizing a proactive mindset towards health and recovery can empower individuals to take control of their aging journey, enabling them to navigate the challenges of injury while continuing to build strength and resilience in their later years.

How To Prevent Frailty

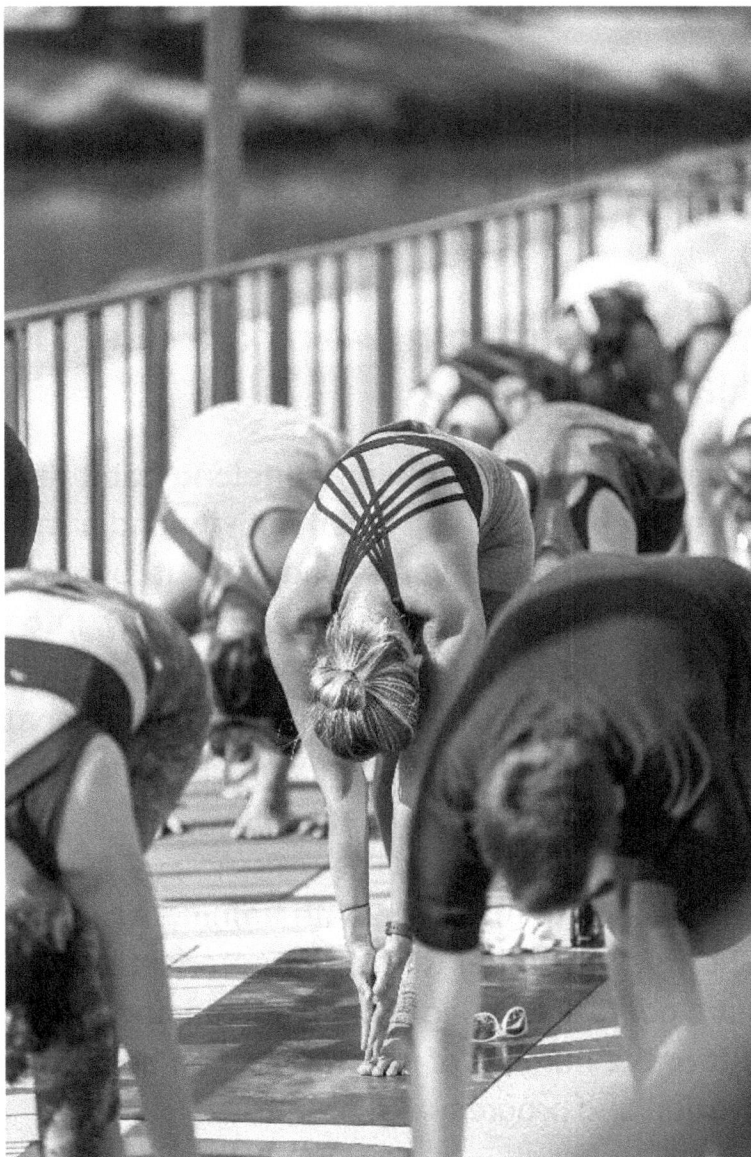

Chapter 10

Maintaining Long-Term Strength and Health

Making Strength Training a Lifelong Habit

Making strength training a lifelong habit requires a commitment to both physical activity and a mindset geared toward health and longevity. It begins with establishing a routine that fits seamlessly into your daily life. This might mean scheduling specific times each week for workouts, choosing convenient locations such as home or a nearby gym, and ensuring that your environment is conducive to exercise.

The key is to make strength training a regular part of your lifestyle, rather than a temporary effort. Setting realistic goals, such as gradually increasing the weight you lift or the number of repetitions, can help maintain motivation and progress.

Incorporating variety into your strength training regimen is essential to prevent boredom and promote adherence. Mixing different exercises, using various equipment, or trying out new classes can keep the workouts fresh and engaging.

Additionally, incorporating functional movements that mimic everyday activities helps reinforce the importance of strength training in daily life. This approach not only enhances motivation but also provides practical benefits that translate into improved overall health and reduced risk of frailty.

Social support plays a significant role in making strength training a lifelong habit. Engaging in group classes or working out with friends can create a sense of community and accountability. Sharing your goals and progress with others fosters encouragement, making it easier to stay committed.

Whether through informal partnerships or joining fitness groups, having a support system can significantly enhance your dedication to regular strength training.

Tracking progress is another effective strategy for maintaining motivation over time. Keeping a journal of your workouts, noting the weights lifted, repetitions completed, and changes in your physical abilities can provide tangible evidence of your improvements.

This not only inspires continued effort but also allows for adjustments in your training program as needed. Celebrating milestones, no matter how small, reinforces the habit and encourages a focus on long-term benefits.

Lastly, it is crucial to listen to your body and adjust your approach as you age. Flexibility in your routine ensures that you remain engaged and safe in your strength training endeavors. Recognizing when to modify exercises or reduce intensity can prevent injury and promote longevity in your training practices.

By prioritizing both strength and safety, you can cultivate a sustainable habit that supports your overall health and helps prevent frailty as you age.

Adapting Your Routine as You Age

As individuals age, their bodies undergo various physiological changes that can affect strength, balance, and overall health. Adapting your routine to accommodate these changes is crucial in preventing frailty.

This adaptation involves modifying exercise regimens, dietary habits, and daily activities to maintain independence and enhance quality of life. Recognizing that what worked in earlier years may no longer be effective is the first step toward creating a sustainable routine that promotes vitality.

Strength training should remain a cornerstone of any fitness routine, but the approach may need to shift as one ages. Incorporating lighter weights with higher repetitions can be beneficial for building endurance and maintaining muscle mass without risking injury. Additionally, focusing on functional movements that mimic daily activities—such as squatting, lifting, and reaching—can improve balance and stability. Engaging in activities like yoga or Pilates can also enhance flexibility and core strength, which are essential for preventing falls and maintaining mobility.

Nutrition plays a pivotal role in combating frailty. As metabolism slows down with age, dietary adjustments may be necessary to ensure adequate nutrient intake. Emphasizing whole foods rich in protein, vitamins, and minerals can help maintain muscle mass and overall health. I

ncluding sources of healthy fats, such as avocados and nuts, along with plenty of fruits and vegetables, supports immune function and reduces inflammation. Staying hydrated is equally important, as dehydration can lead to fatigue and decreased muscle function.

Incorporating regular health check-ups into your routine is essential as you age. These visits can help identify potential health issues early on and allow for timely interventions. Working with healthcare providers to monitor conditions such as hypertension, diabetes, or osteoporosis can lead to tailored recommendations that fit your lifestyle. Furthermore, discussing any new exercise or dietary changes with a physician or a registered dietitian can ensure that your adaptations are safe and effective.

Lastly, mental health and social engagement are integral to preventing frailty. Establishing a routine that includes social interaction, whether through group exercises, community events, or simply spending time with friends and family, can bolster emotional well-being and reduce feelings of isolation.

Engaging in hobbies, learning new skills, or volunteering can also provide a sense of purpose and fulfillment. By nurturing both physical and mental health, individuals can create a balanced routine that supports a robust and active lifestyle well into their later years.

The Future of Aging: Trends in Strength and Health

As the population continues to age, the concept of aging is evolving beyond the traditional narrative of decline and frailty. Instead, there is a growing emphasis on strength and health as key components of successful aging. This shift in perspective is driven by advancements in research, a greater understanding of the aging process, and an increasing number of individuals who prioritize their health and fitness as they grow older.

The future of aging will likely see a more proactive approach to maintaining physical strength, which is essential for preventing frailty and promoting overall well-being.

One significant trend in the future of aging is the integration of technology into health and fitness routines. Wearable devices and health applications are making it easier for older adults to track their physical activity, monitor vital signs, and receive personalized fitness guidance.

These tools can help individuals set and achieve fitness goals, making it easier to incorporate strength training and other forms of exercise into their daily lives. As technology continues to evolve, we can expect even more innovative solutions that cater specifically to the needs of older adults, empowering them to take control of their health.

Another trend is the increased focus on community and social connections as vital components of health in aging. Research has consistently shown that social engagement and support significantly impact physical and mental health.

Programs that promote group exercise, community health initiatives, and social activities can help older adults stay active and connected, reducing the risk of frailty. The future will likely see more community-based efforts aimed at fostering connections among older adults, encouraging a holistic approach to health that includes both physical and social well-being.

Nutrition will also play a crucial role in the future of aging. As awareness grows about the connection between diet and health outcomes, there is likely to be a greater emphasis on nutrition tailored to the needs of older adults. Diets rich in protein, essential vitamins, and minerals will be highlighted as vital for maintaining muscle mass and overall strength.

Additionally, educational programs will emerge to teach older adults about the importance of nutrition in preventing frailty, equipping them with the knowledge to make informed dietary choices that support their health.

Finally, the future of aging will witness a paradigm shift in how society views older adults. As more individuals embrace active lifestyles and challenge stereotypes about aging, there will be a cultural movement towards celebrating strength and vitality in later life. This shift will encourage older adults to prioritize their health and fitness, reducing the stigma associated with aging and frailty.

By fostering an environment that values strength and well-being, we can create a society where aging is seen not as a decline but as an opportunity for growth, resilience, and continued contribution to the community.

How To Prevent Frailty

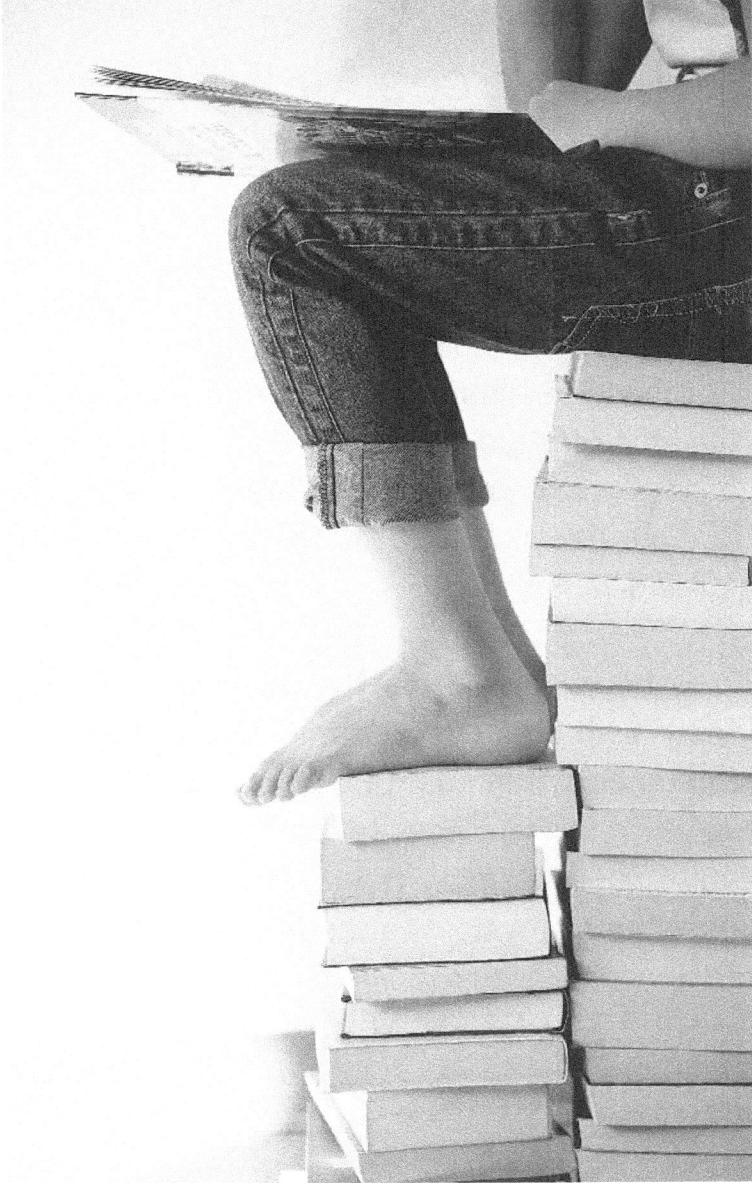

Chapter 11

Resources for Further Learning

Recommended Books and Articles

For those seeking to prevent frailty as they age, a wealth of literature exists that provides valuable insights into strength-building and overall wellness. One notable title is "The Science of Strength Training" by Dr. David W. Hill.

This book delves into the physiological changes that occur with aging and emphasizes the importance of resistance training. Dr. Hill outlines effective strategies and routines tailored for older adults, making it an essential read for anyone looking to enhance their physical strength and combat age-related decline.

Another significant resource is "Strong Women Stay Young" by Dr. Miriam E. Nelson. This book specifically focuses on women and their unique health challenges as they age. Dr. Nelson combines research with practical exercises, nutritional advice, and motivational tips, empowering readers to take charge of their health.

The emphasis on strength training as a means to improve bone density and muscle mass makes this book a key reference for individuals aiming to prevent frailty.

In addition to these books, scholarly articles provide a more in-depth understanding of frailty and its prevention. The article "Physical Activity and Frailty in Older Adults" published in the Journal of Aging and Physical Activity reviews numerous studies that link regular physical activity to reduced frailty risk. It highlights the types of exercises most beneficial for older adults and encourages a proactive approach to maintaining physical fitness.

This article serves as a valuable resource for those interested in evidence-based practices for frailty prevention.

Online platforms also offer a plethora of articles and blogs dedicated to aging and strength training. Websites like the National Institute on Aging feature articles that discuss the importance of nutrition, social engagement, and exercise in promoting health as one ages. These resources are accessible and provide practical tips that can be easily integrated into daily life, making them ideal for individuals looking to adopt a holistic approach to frailty prevention.

Lastly, joining a community or reading group focused on aging and health can enhance motivation and provide additional resources. Many local libraries and community centers host book clubs centered around health and wellness themes.

Engaging with others who share similar goals can inspire commitment and accountability, making the journey toward strength and vitality more enjoyable. By exploring these recommended books and articles, individuals can equip themselves with the knowledge and tools necessary to prevent frailty and embrace healthier aging.

Online Courses and Videos

Online courses and videos have become invaluable resources for individuals seeking to prevent frailty as they age. With the increasing reliance on digital platforms, accessing information about strength training, nutrition, and overall wellness has never been easier.

These resources cater to various learning styles, allowing users to engage with material at their own pace and convenience. From comprehensive courses offered by fitness experts to short instructional videos on specific exercises, the online world is rich with content aimed at promoting physical health and resilience.

One of the primary advantages of online courses is their accessibility. People can participate from the comfort of their homes, removing barriers such as transportation and time constraints. Many platforms offer courses tailored specifically to older adults, focusing on safe and effective exercises that enhance strength, balance, and flexibility.

This is particularly important for individuals who may feel intimidated by traditional gym settings. Online courses provide a supportive environment where learners can build their confidence and gradually progress in their fitness journeys.

In addition to strength training, online resources often cover essential aspects of nutrition and healthy living. Many courses include modules on dietary recommendations, meal planning, and maintaining a balanced diet as one ages.

Understanding the nutritional needs specific to older adults is crucial in preventing frailty. Video tutorials can also demonstrate healthy cooking techniques and quick meal prep ideas, making it easier for individuals to adopt healthier eating habits. The combination of exercise and nutrition education is key in fostering a holistic approach to health.

Community engagement is another vital component of online learning. Many platforms offer forums or groups where participants can share their experiences, ask questions, and motivate one another. This sense of community can provide emotional support and accountability, which are essential for long-term adherence to a fitness regimen.

Additionally, some courses incorporate live sessions or Q&A opportunities with instructors, allowing for direct interaction and personalized guidance.

Such connections can enhance the learning experience and encourage participants to stay committed to their health goals.

Finally, the wealth of online resources allows for continuous learning and adaptation. As individuals progress in their fitness levels, they can easily find advanced courses or specialized content that aligns with their evolving needs. This flexibility ensures that users remain engaged and challenged, which is crucial in preventing the stagnation that can lead to frailty.

By leveraging the extensive array of online courses and videos, individuals can take proactive steps toward building strength and maintaining their health as they age, ultimately leading to a more vibrant and active lifestyle.

Local Community Resources and Programs

Local community resources and programs play a crucial role in preventing frailty among older adults. These resources are designed to provide support, education, and activities that promote physical health, mental well-being, and social engagement. By accessing these programs, individuals can enhance their quality of life, improve their physical resilience, and build a supportive network that fosters independence and vitality.

One of the most valuable resources available in many communities is senior centers. These centers offer a variety of activities, from fitness classes tailored to older adults to social events that encourage interaction.

Participating in regular exercise can help maintain strength, balance, and flexibility, all of which are essential in preventing frailty. Additionally, many senior centers provide educational workshops on nutrition, health management, and other relevant topics, empowering individuals with knowledge to make informed choices about their health.

Local health departments and community health organizations also provide a wealth of resources aimed at preventing frailty. These organizations often offer free or low-cost health screenings, vaccinations, and wellness programs.

Regular health check-ups can help identify potential health issues before they become serious, ensuring that older adults receive timely interventions.

Additionally, many health departments run initiatives focused on healthy eating and physical activity, which are critical components of maintaining strength and preventing frailty.

Another important aspect of community resources is the availability of support groups and social clubs. These groups can significantly impact mental health by reducing feelings of isolation and loneliness, which are common among older adults. Engaging with peers in shared activities fosters a sense of belonging and encourages individuals to stay active.

Many communities also have volunteer programs that allow seniors to contribute their time and skills, further enhancing their sense of purpose and connectedness to the community.

Finally, it is essential for individuals to explore local transportation options that facilitate access to these resources. Many communities offer transportation services specifically for seniors, making it easier for them to attend fitness classes, health screenings, and social events.

By utilizing these services, older adults can maintain their independence and remain integrated within their communities, all of which are vital in preventing frailty. By taking advantage of local resources and programs, individuals can actively engage in their health and well-being as they age.

Author Notes & Acknowledgments

First and foremost, I would like to express my deepest gratitude to the people who inspired and supported me throughout the journey of writing this book. This project would not have been possible without their unwavering belief in me and their invaluable contributions.

To my wife, thank you for your constant encouragement and understanding. Your love and support have been my anchor during the challenging times of researching and writing this book. Your belief in my ability to make a difference in people's lives has been my driving force.

I would also like to disclose that this book contains some renewed artificial intelligence-generated content. I really appreciate very recent technological innovation by outstanding scientists and of course our reader's understanding.

Lastly, I want to express my deepest gratitude to the readers of this book. I sincerely hope the strategies and methods outlined within these pages will provide you with the knowledge and tools needed to truly make your life much better. Your commitment to seeking any good solutions and willingness to explore multiple methods is commendable.

Author Bio

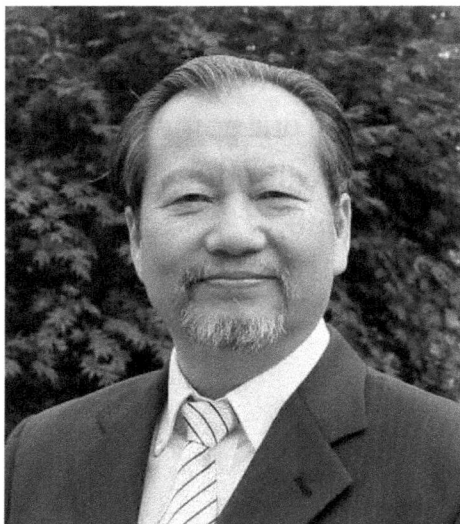

Johnson Wu earned his MD in 1982. With over 40 years of clinical experience, he has worked in hospitals in Zhejiang and Shanghai, China, as well as the Royal Marsden Hospital (part of Imperial College) in London, UK. Upon the recommendation of Sir Aaron Klug, the president of The Royal Society and a Nobel Prize winner in Chemistry, Dr. Wu was honorably awarded a British Royal Society Fellowship. He has published over 100 medical books in many countries and currently practices medicine in Canada.

www.ingramcontent.com/pod-product-compliance
Lightning Source LLC
Chambersburg PA
CBHW060244030426

42335CB00014B/1589